ETERNAL VITALITY

A Scientific Odyssey to Age Defying Wellness

James R. Persinger

ETERNAL VITALITY

ETERNAL VITALITY

INTRODUCTION

The Aging Process Unveiled

CHAPTER ONE

HEREDITARY QUALITIES AND MATURING

Grasping Hereditary Impacts

Role of DNA in Maturing

CHAPTER TWO

SUSTENANCE AND LIFE SPAN

Effect of Diet on Maturing

Superfoods for Better Maturing

CHAPTER THREE

ACTIVITY AND MATURING

The Job of Actual work

Fitting Activity for Aging Great

CHAPTER FOUR

MENTAL WELLBEING

Keeping up with Smartness

Systems for Mental Health

CHAPTER FIVE

REST AND MATURING

Significance of Value Rest

ETERNAL VITALITY

Rest Cleanliness for Ideal Maturing

CHAPTER SIX

WAY OF LIFE ELEMENTS

Pressure The board

Social Associations and Aging

CONCLUSION

ETERNAL VITALITY

ETERNAL VITALITY

INTRODUCTION

The Aging Process Unveiled

From birth to death, aging involves changes in one's physical, social, psychological, and spiritual well-being. Albeit maturing is a continuous cycle, the benefit of maturing is seen distinctively at various places all the while. A portion of the progressions are expected with euphoria, like a child's most memorable tooth or initial step. Different changes are welcomed with a more negative reaction, for example, taking out the main silver hairs that show up. Youth is esteemed in American culture; while indications of maturing are concealed with face-lifts, wrinkle creams, and hair colors.

ETERNAL VITALITY

When youthful attractiveness begins to change, the process of physical maturation that is so eagerly anticipated in the early stages of life is viewed very negatively. As a result of these prevalent attitudes, people deny the signs of aging. A few people quit commending birthday events after a specific age. The cliché view of maturing as a time of disintegration and decline are consequently sustained. The positive parts of maturing are overlooked. Each phase of life has its own pluses and minuses. At times in advanced age, the equilibrium might appear to tip to additional negatives than up-sides, however this isn't because of the regular maturing process. There are numerous positive parts of maturing. Following 70 or 80 years of living, people will generally have a reasonable feeling of their qualities and needs. More seasoned people can go with unequivocal decisions about how to utilize their significant investment. Their needs might be altogether different from what guardians, family, or companions maintain that they should be. People who are older have acquired methods for adjusting to changes; they have figured out how to get by. Old age can carry an opportunity to talk one's viewpoint. Due to retirement, numerous more established people have more noteworthy opportunity to seek after interests, to utilize time to think and to reflect. Jung said that as we get older, we become more like ourselves. The high level phases of maturing are a typical, normal piece of actual development. It may be more productive to accept life's changes without fear or denial rather than placing such a high value on youth.

Characteristics of Older People As a long-term care ombudsman (LTCO), you will interact with older people, their families, and the people who take care of them. You must comprehend the "big picture" of the senior population, which is defined here as individuals 65 years of age or older, in order to better comprehend the population of long-term care residents on which you are primarily focused. Who then are the elderly? At what age does an individual age significantly? Has that person changed when they go to bed at 64 and wake up at 65 the next morning? Ordered age doesn't necessarily in all cases relate to an individual's sentiments. Albeit an individual might be eighty years of age, the ! Asset Material The Maturing System 2 man might feel like he/she is forty. The age an individual feels might change with the hour of day, the day of the week, or potentially exercises or stresses present in such individual's reality. An individual might be exceptionally vivacious on Saturday, yet extremely drained and sluggish on Monday morning. Realizing an individual's sequential age informs you barely anything concerning

ETERNAL VITALITY

that singular's sentiments or capacities. In any case, in this country, we sort people by ordered age. The senior population, or people 65 and older, is described in detail in the following key statistics1.

CHAPTER ONE
HEREDITARY QUALITIES AND MATURING

Grasping Hereditary Impacts

The sizable hereditary impacts on individual contrasts in weakness to creating reliance on a drug (see underneath) are probably going to cover considerably with by and large hereditary effects on capacities to stop, as well likewise with hereditary effects on various related aggregates and comorbid conditions. At a sub-atomic level, this implies that DNA succession variations that are passed from one age to another can, in lenient conditions, work to modify these weaknesses. As a result, we can begin by providing an overview of the kinds of DNA variants that may contribute to these vulnerabilities. We incorporate novel information for potential jobs for duplicate number variations (CNVs). The topic of shared genetic influences on co morbidities and their possible implications for thinking about, treating, and preventing addiction is then advanced to the next level.

It had never been thought that PD was influenced by genes. However, in recent decades, specific gene mutations in familial forms of Parkinson's disease have been identified, and these findings may provide us with important insights into the idiopathic condition's pathophysiology. Most broadly examined have been changes in α-syncline. Misfolding of the protein is caused by pathogenic forms of -synuclein, which is analogous to the misfolding that is associated with amyloid plaques in Alzheimer's disease. Various other hereditary types of the infection have been clarified, like those including leucine-rich recurrent kinase 2 (LRRK2), DJ-1, which might be an abnormal peroxiredoxin-like peroxidase, and parkin. Like α-synuclein, parkin, and ubiquitin-3-ligase, can total in cells. Parkin ubiquitinates itself advancing its own debasement, and familial transformations of parkin with decreased ubiquitin ligase movement evoke the conglomerations of Lewy bodies. These Lewy bodies incorporate α-synuclein, parkin, and synphilin. Mice, drosophila, and C. elegans containing freak types of these qualities have given significant models to PD research. Evaluation of the misfolding of proteins in Parkinson's disease and other conditions has been made easier with yeast.

Role of DNA in Maturing

Maturing is a perplexing, diverse interaction prompting inescapable useful downfall influencing each organ and tissue. Surprisingly, it is at this point unclear in the event that maturing has a bringing together causal system or is grounded in different sources. Phenotypically, the maturing system is related with a wide assortment of highlights at the sub-atomic, cell and physiological level, e.g., genomic and epigenomic modifications, loss of proteostasis, declining in general cell and sub-cell capability, liberation of flagging frameworks. Be that as it may, the relative significance, robotic interrelationships and various leveled request of those maturing highlights have not been explained. Here, we blend collecting proof that DNA harm influences the overwhelming majority of parts of the maturing aggregate making it a most probable binding together reason for maturing. Consequently, focusing on DNA harm and its robotic connections with the maturing aggregate will give a legitimate reasoning to creating mediations to balance age-related brokenness and illness in show.

Every day, the respectability and steadiness of DNA are tested by exogenous physical, substance, or natural specialists, as well as by endogenous cycles, including DNA replication botches, unconstrained hydrolytic responses, and receptive oxygen species (ROS). In this way, contingent upon the wellspring of harm, DNA can be impacted in various ways, including nucleotide modifications, cumbersome adducts, single-strand breaks (SSB), and twofold strand breaks (DSB). To battle dangers presented by DNA harm, cells have advanced complex and finely controlled systems altogether alluded to as DNA harm reaction (DDR) which distinguishes DNA injuries, flags their presence, and advances their maintenance [22, 23, 24]. Notwithstanding, concurring with the genome upkeep speculation of maturing, DNA fix might itself at any point be likely to progress in years related changes and disintegration, permitting aggregation of harms (Figure 2). The wide variety of DNA-sore sorts requires various, to a great extent unmistakable DNA fix systems that vary in their parts, though a few injuries are likely to coordinate protein-interceded inversion, most are fixed by a grouping of synergist occasions intervened by numerous proteins [22]. As a result, it has been demonstrated that the accumulation of mutations and epimutations that eventually lead to cell dysfunction, senescence, or apoptosis in cells with defects in key DDR proteins accelerates the aging process.

CHAPTER TWO
SUSTENANCE AND LIFE SPAN

Effect of Diet on Maturing

Research demonstrates the way that eating super handled food sources can accelerate the maturing of your phones. Quite a bit of this is because of super handled food sources frequently containing a high measure of hydrogenated oils, which are loaded with trans fats and can advance the persistent irritation that hurries the breakdown (or maturing) of your phones.

ETERNAL VITALITY

As anyone might expect, all Blue Zone eats less put accentuation on genuine food utilization: crude, cooked, ground, or matured — with recipes that convey a fixing rundown of six things or less, a sign of approval for the idea that food, not pills or business drinks, is the best wellspring of supplements.

Go nuts are a great whole-food snack to replace more processed, unhealthy snacks that can accelerate the natural process of gaining weight as we get older. A special reward of these forces to be reckoned with is that nuts loaded with omega-3 unsaturated fats might have the option to further develop concentration and abatement the gamble of Alzheimer's sickness.

ETERNAL VITALITY

Be innovative with your calcium and fiber sources

Calcium keeps up with bone strength and keep bones sound during more established age, while fiber can assist with decreasing the gamble of Type 2 diabetes and coronary illness — and both are key supplements to remember for your eating routine as you age.

However, this does not necessarily imply that the solution is to rush out and buy special drinks and chews that are frequently advertised to adults of a certain age. For a calcium-rich lift, incorporate dairy items like milk, cheddar, or yogurt in your dinners. What's more, in the event that dairy processing is an issue, check goat's milk variants of these items out; they're frequently thought to be more straightforward to process. On the off chance that dairy isn't your thing, an astonishing measure of calcium can be covered through plant-based food sources like seeds, beans and lentils, and salad greens. A reward: these food sources can carry out twofold responsibility in giving calcium, yet a sound portion of fiber too, which can support processing and satiation and assist with cutting LDL (otherwise called "terrible" cholesterol).

Remain hydrated

ETERNAL VITALITY

A basic yet imperative player in one's wellbeing, water is required for pretty much every physical process including assimilation, keeping up with internal heat level, and course. Nonetheless, what many don't understand is that the body loses water as we age — and alongside that, tragically, we likewise lose our feeling of thirst. To battle this misfortune, taste on water over the course of the day, going for the gold. Or on the other hand, in the event that you like to stir up your fluids, cell reinforcement rich green tea may likewise improve memory and mental sharpness as you age.

Espresso and red wine with some restraint

ETERNAL VITALITY

Control is key here; be that as it may, both espresso and red wine can assume a free part in a sound eating regimen for maturing grown-ups. Both cherished refreshments contain cancer prevention agents, which are known to help the resistant framework. Likewise, these drinks are known to advance blood stream and might actually increment life length. As well as being great for you, there are likewise feel-great advantages to both espresso and red wine. Some exploration shows that both could assume a part in assisting with lessening the gamble of sadness, and caffeine has been explored to work couple with a compound in espresso to support cerebrum wellbeing and possibly assist with forestalling mind illnesses like Alzheimer's.

Abstain from gorging and think about irregular fasting

As we age, our digestion eases back — an interaction that probably begins as soon as the age of 40. While smart dieting and exercise propensities embraced early can assist with combatting weight gain related with this dialing back of our framework, another choice is to be more aware of when, and how, you structure your caloric admission. Proof is collecting that eating in a 6-hour time frame and fasting for 18 hours (regularly referred to now as discontinuous fasting) can set off a metabolic change from glucose-based to ketone-based energy, with expanded pressure opposition, expanded life span, and a diminished rate of illnesses, including malignant growth and corpulence. Blue Zone populaces will frequently eat their biggest feast from the beginning in the day (known as their "break quick" dinner) and will direct food utilization as they advance toward the night hours, when the body, and digestion, normally starts to dial back.

Superfoods for Better Maturing

Superfoods are not a particular food classification all alone. Rather, this chivalrous sounding name essentially portrays entire, negligibly handled food sources that are supplement thick. For the most part, superfoods contain sound fats, nutrients, minerals, cell reinforcements, and different mixtures found to advance great wellbeing and forestall sickness and infection. While most are plant-based, certain fish and dairy items may likewise be considered superfoods.

What superfoods should seniors eat? No single superfood gives all the sustenance more seasoned grown-ups need. That is the reason, assuming you're really focusing on a friend or family member, you'll need to urge them to eat a wide assortment of nutritious food sources day to day.

Are there against maturing superfoods?

ETERNAL VITALITY

What food varieties are considered superfoods? There are numerous — however here are some superfood rockstars known to add to solid maturing.

Carotenoids, found in dark-colored leafy greens like spinach and kale, have been shown to protect the eyes from oxidative damage. Spinach is likewise stacked with nutrients An and C, which assist with safeguarding the heart and moderate pulse levels. Vitamin K is another verdant green supplement, found to assume a significant part in forestalling osteoporosis. Mixed greens are tasty in a plate of mixed greens, in a sandwich, or sautéed with a sprinkle of solid oil.

ETERNAL VITALITY

Spinach, kale, collard greens, broccoli and other salad greens can make drugs to forestall blood clumps less viable. Green verdant veggies are plentiful in vitamin K, which collaborates with the normal blood-diminishing medication warfarin (brand name Coumadin). Kindly talk with your primary care physician prior to adding more mixed greens to your eating routine.

Cruciferous vegetables

This veggie family incorporates broccoli, cabbage, Brussels fledglings, and turnips — which are all extraordinary wellsprings of fiber, nutrients, and malignant growth forestalling phytochemicals. Cruciferous vegetables are scrumptious and incredibly adaptable. Throw them in soups, pasta dishes, and goulashes; steam them; or stir-fry them with olive oil and some seasoning.

Blueberries

In a meeting with U.S. News and World Report, Reema Kanda, an enrolled dietitian nutritionist with the Hoag Muscular Establishment in Irvine, California, says concentrates on show that blueberries have positive neurocognitive impacts in the two creatures and people. According to therefore, Kanda, they might assist with postponing age-related mental deterioration.

ETERNAL VITALITY

Blueberries are likewise wealthy in cancer prevention agents, intensifies that assist with safeguarding our cells against free-extremist harm and decrease the gamble for coronary illness and malignant growth. These delightful, adaptable berries can be added to smoothies and treats, sprinkled over oat, and obviously, eaten without help from anyone else!

Nuts and seeds, such as hazelnuts, pistachios, almonds, and pecans, are loaded with antioxidants, fiber, and plant protein. Additionally, they contain monounsaturated fats, which are believed to lower the risk of heart disease. However long the more established grown-up you care for has no known sensitivities, nuts make a tasty independent tidbit. They can likewise be mixed into pestos or utilized as a delightful serving of mixed greens clincher.

Seeds are another wonderful superfood. A recent report found that chia seeds — wealthy in omega-3 unsaturated fats, fiber, and cell reinforcements — may assist with forestalling malignant growth and safeguard the heart and liver. Other delicious seed choices incorporate hemp seed and flax seed, which are likewise high in irritation battling omega-3 unsaturated fats.

Considerations regarding nuts and seeds: They are high in fat and calories, so restricting utilization to a little modest bunch every day is ideal.

Eggs

Eggs have been a wellspring of dietary contention over the course of the years because of cholesterol tracked down in the yolk. However, elderly people may be deficient in important nutrients like selenium, vitamin D, and vitamin B12. Egg yolks likewise contain choline, a supplement and synapse liable for controlling temperament and memory.

Salmon

Greasy fish (e.g., salmon, herring, mackerel, trout, and fish steak) is a brilliant wellspring of protein — a supplement crucial to keeping up with bulk in more seasoned grown-ups. Additionally, it is high in omega-3 fatty acids, which have been shown to lower the risk of heart disease. An extraordinary method for partaking in a new fish filet is to gently prepare it, heat it, and present with a side of cruciferous vegetables.

Plain Greek yogurt

With regards to protein, Greek yogurt conveys. Only one cup has 17 grams of protein as well as 20% of the day to day suggested admission of calcium. Another reason Greek yogurt is regarded as one of the best superfoods for seniors is this: It contains probiotics, which assist us with keeping up with stomach wellbeing. Probiotics have been displayed to help with absorption, support invulnerable capability, and even forestall contamination.

Greek yogurt, plain and unsweetened, is extremely adaptable. It tends to be finished off with granola and berries or even be fill in for sharp cream in specific recipes. Look for yogurt without added sugar that is made with whole milk or reduced-fat milk.

Avocados

Avocado is a dietary force to be reckoned with, stacked with sustaining fats, cell reinforcements, and different supplements that help head-to-toe wellbeing. This smooth finished natural product is tasty in guacamole or spread on toast. On the off chance that the more established grown-up you care for could do without the flavor of avocado, think about mixing it into a natural product smoothie for an unobtrusive nourishing lift.

CHAPTER THREE
ACTIVITY AND MATURING

The Job of Actual work

As a more established grown-up, normal active work is quite possibly of the main thing you can accomplish for your wellbeing. It can forestall or postpone a significant number of the medical issues that appear to accompany age. It moreover helps your muscles with growing further so you can keep on doing your ordinary activities without becoming subject to others.

Remember, some actual work is superior to none by any stretch of the imagination. Your

ETERNAL VITALITY

medical advantages will likewise increment with the more active work that you do.

Grown-ups matured 65 and more established need:

Something like 150 minutes every week (for instance, 30 minutes per day, 5 days per seven day stretch) of moderate-power movement like lively strolling. Or on the other hand they need 75 minutes per seven day stretch of enthusiastic force action like climbing, running, or running.

No less than 2 days every seven day stretch of exercises that reinforce muscles.

Furthermore exercises to further develop balance, like remaining on one foot.

ETERNAL VITALITY

In the event that persistent circumstances influence your capacity to meet these suggestions, be basically as actually dynamic as your capacities and conditions permit.

Walking

Moderate-force vigorous movement

(like energetic strolling) for 150 minutes (for instance, 30 minutes per day, 5 days every week)

Power lifting

Muscle-fortifying exercises

on at least 2 days every week that work all significant muscle gatherings (legs, hips, back, mid-region, chest, shoulders, and arms).

ETERNAL VITALITY

Balance

Balance exercises

Strolling heel-to-toe or remaining from a sitting position.

Running

Enthusiastic force vigorous action

(like running or running) for 75 minutes (1 hour and 15 minutes) consistently

Fitting Activity for Aging Great

Ways to tailor Wellness Techniques for More seasoned Grown-ups

Begin Without rushing: In the event that you're new to practice or returning after a break, slip into it. Start with low-influence practices and slowly increment force.

Training for Strength: Consolidate opposition groups, light loads, or bodyweight activities to assemble bulk and keep up with bone thickness.

Workouts for Flexibility: Yoga and Pilates are excellent options for enhancing core strength, balance, and flexibility.

Cardio is Vital: Cardiovascular activities, even lively strolling or moving, can further develop heart wellbeing and perseverance.

Pay attention to Your Body: Pay attention to how you feel in your body. It's fundamental to separate between great agony (like muscle irritation) and awful torment (like joint distress or sharp torments).

Remain Hydrated: We lose the ability to feel thirsty as we get older. Guarantee you're drinking adequate water, particularly after exercises.

Counsel Experts: Before beginning any new exercise routine, always consult with medical professionals.

Making Wellness a Party

One of the most outstanding ways of remaining inspired is by making wellness a social movement:

ETERNAL VITALITY

Join a gym or fitness class: Numerous rec centers offer classes explicitly intended for more seasoned grown-ups.

Stroll with Companions: Strolling clubs can offer both social communication and exercise.

Try workouts with a partner: Practices that require an accomplice can be both tomfoolery and testing.

ETERNAL VITALITY

CHAPTER FOUR
MENTAL WELLBEING

Keeping up with Smartness

Everybody has an intermittent "senior second." Perhaps you've gone into the kitchen and can't recollect why, or can't remember a recognizable name during a discussion. Memory omissions can happen at whatever stage in life, yet maturing alone is by and large not a reason for mental deterioration. At the point when critical cognitive decline happens among more established individuals, it is by and large not because of maturing however to

ETERNAL VITALITY

natural problems, cerebrum injury, or neurological disease.

Studies have demonstrated the way that you can assist with forestalling mental degradation and diminish the gamble of dementia with some essential great wellbeing propensities:

remaining actually dynamic

getting sufficient rest

not smoking

having great social associations

restricting liquor to something like one beverage daily

Eating a Mediterranean style diet.

ETERNAL VITALITY

Memory and other mental changes can be disappointing, yet fortunately, on account of many years of exploration, you can figure out how to get your brain dynamic. There are different procedures we can use to assist with keeping up with mental wellness. The following are a few you could attempt.

Shield yourself from the harm of persistent aggravation.

Science has shown the way that consistent, inferior bothering can change into a peaceful killer that adds to cardiovas-cular sickness, dangerous development, type 2 diabetes and various conditions. Get straightforward tips to

ETERNAL VITALITY

battle aggravation and remain sound - - from Harvard Clinical School specialists.

Continue your education

A higher level of education is linked to improved mental health in later life. Specialists believe that high level training might assist with keeping areas of strength for memory getting an individual into the propensity for being intellectually dynamic. Testing your mind with mental activity is accepted to initiate processes that assist with keeping up with individual synapses and animate correspondence among them. Numerous people have occupations that keep them mentally unique. Chasing after a side interest, mastering another expertise, chipping in or coaching are extra ways of keeping your brain sharp.

 Utilize every one of your faculties

The more detects you use in picking up something, there a greater amount of your mind that will be engaged with holding the memory. In one review, grown-ups were shown a progression of smell-went with, genuinely unbiased pictures. They were not drawn nearer to review what they saw. They were then shown a set of images, this time without smells, and asked which ones they had previously seen. They had amazing review for all scent matched pictures, and particularly for those related with wonderful scents. Mind imaging demonstrated that the piriform cortex, the principal scent handling locale of the cerebrum, became dynamic when individuals saw protests initially matched with scents, despite the fact that the scents were at this point not present and the subjects hadn't attempted to recollect them. So challenge every one of your faculties as you adventure into the new.

Have confidence in yourself

A poor memory can be exacerbated by myths about growing up. Moderately aged and more established students do more terrible on memory assignments when they're presented to negative generalizations about maturing and memory, and better when the messages are certain about memory safeguarding into advanced age. Individuals who accept that they are not in charge of their memory capability — kidding about "senior minutes" over and over again, maybe — are less inclined to work at keeping up with or further developing their memory abilities and accordingly are bound to encounter mental deterioration. Assuming you accept you can improve and you make an interpretation of that conviction into training, you have a superior possibility keeping your psyche sharp.

Focus on your cerebrum use

ETERNAL VITALITY

On the off chance that you don't have to utilize mental energy recalling where you laid your keys or the hour of your granddaughter's birthday celebration, you'll be better ready to focus on learning and recollecting new and significant things. Exploit advanced cell updates, schedules and organizers, maps, shopping records, document envelopes, and address books to keep routine data available. Dole out a spot at home for your glasses, sack, keys, and various things you use regularly.

Write down or repeat what you want to remember

Space it out When timed correctly

repetition is most effective as a learning tool. It's best not to rehash something ordinarily in a brief period, as though you were packing for a test. Taking everything into account, re-focus on the essentials after logically longer time spans — when an hour, then, similar to precision, then, reliably. Scattering times of study further develops memory and is especially significant when you are attempting to dominate muddled data, like the subtleties of another work task.

Systems for Mental Health

So how would you keep your cerebrum solid, remain intellectually fit, and fabricate your mental save? It's simpler for certain individuals than for other people. Also, however hereditary qualities set up for your cerebrum wellbeing, you can effectively further develop your mind wellbeing and mental wellness.

First it is essential to recollect that you want a solid body to have a sound cerebrum. Consequently, guaranteeing your mind wellbeing relies on consistently seeing your primary care physician, following her or his suggestions, and dealing with any medical issue you have.

The core of our cerebrum wellbeing and mental work out regime, in any case, includes way of life changes. Six pillars have been identified by Harvard Medical School researchers as essential to any successful program for cognitive fitness and brain health. Despite the fact that we refer to them as "steps," they should all be completed simultaneously:

Step 1: Step 2: Follow a plant-based diet. Work-out consistently

Stage 3: Get adequate rest Step 4: Deal with your pressure

Stage 5: Sustain social contacts

Stage 6: Keep on testing your cerebrum

Together, these can yield genuine outcomes, prompting changes in both your cerebrum's construction and capability. In any case, the catchphrase is "together." These elements are equivalent pieces of a firm arrangement — they don't work in disengagement. Essentially eating more fiber or adding a morning stroll to your routine isn't sufficient to thwart cognitive deterioration. Instead, results are achieved through a combination of exercise, diet, sleep, stress management, social interaction, and mental stimulation.

CHAPTER FIVE
REST AND MATURING

Significance of Value Rest

Consistently dozing under seven hours around evening time can seriously jeopardize your wellbeing and security, which is the reason it's

ETERNAL VITALITY

fundamental that you focus on and safeguard your rest consistently.

Getting a pleasant evening's rest is stunningly critical for your prosperity. As a matter of fact, it's similarly basically as significant as eating a reasonable, nutritious eating regimen and working out.

However rest needs change from one individual to another, most grown-ups expect somewhere in the range of 7 and 9 hours of rest each evening. However, up to 35% of grown-ups in the US don't get sufficient rest

May assistance you keep up with or shed pounds

Can further develop fixation and efficiency

ETERNAL VITALITY

Rest is significant for different parts of cerebrum capability.

Can augment athletic execution

May reinforce your heart

Affects sugar digestion and type 2 diabetes risk

Unfortunate rest is connected to sadness

Supports a solid invulnerable framework

Poor rest is connected to expanded irritation

Affects feelings and social cooperations

Rest Cleanliness for Ideal Maturing

As we age, we frequently experience typical changes in our resting designs, for example, becoming sluggish prior, getting up prior, or not dozing as profoundly. Nonetheless, upset rest, awakening tired consistently, and different side effects of sleep deprivation are NOT a typical piece of maturing.

Rest is similarly as essential to your physical and close to home wellbeing as it was the point at which you were more youthful. A decent night's rest further develops focus and memory arrangement, permits your body to fix any phone harm that happened during the day, and revives your safe framework, which thusly assists with forestalling sickness.

More seasoned individuals who don't rest soundly are bound to experience the ill effects of wretchedness, consideration and memory issues, inordinate daytime sluggishness, and experience more evening falls. Deficient rest can likewise prompt serious medical issues, including an expanded gamble of cardiovascular illness, diabetes, weight issues, and bosom disease in ladies.

To work on your nature of rest understanding the fundamental reasons for your rest problems is significant. The accompanying tips can help you distinguish and conquer age-related rest issues, get a decent night's rest, and work on the nature of your cognizant existence.

How much rest do more seasoned grown-ups need?

ETERNAL VITALITY

While rest necessities differ from one individual to another, most solid grown-ups expect seven to nine hours of rest each evening. Notwithstanding, how you feel in the first part of the day is a higher priority than a particular number of hours. Every now and again awakening not feeling rested or feeling tired during the day are the best signs that you're not getting sufficient rest.

How does maturing influence rest?

As you age your body produces lower levels of development chemical, so you'll probably encounter a lessening in sluggish wave or profound rest (a particularly reviving piece of the rest cycle). At the point when this happens you produce less melatonin, importance you'll frequently encounter more divided rest and wake up more frequently during the evening. That is the reason large numbers of us see ourselves as "light sleepers" as we age. You may likewise:

Need to nod off prior at night and get up prior in the first part of the day.

Need to spend longer in bed around evening time to get the long stretches of rest you really want, or make up the deficiency by sleeping during the day.

Tips to further develop rest propensities as you age

ETERNAL VITALITY

As a rule, you can work on your rest by resolving intense subject matters, further developing your rest climate, and picking better daytime propensities.

Since everybody is unique, however, it might take a trial and error to find the particular changes that work best to work on your rest.

Tip 1: Further develop your rest climate

Normally help your melatonin levels. Fake lights around evening time can stifle your body's creation of melatonin, the chemical that makes you languid. Utilize low-wattage bulbs where protected to do as such, and switch off the television and PC something like one hour before bed.

ETERNAL VITALITY

Try not to peruse from an illuminated gadget around evening time (like an iPad). If like to peruse from a tablet or other electronic gadget, change to a Tablet that requires an extra light source.

Ensure your room hushes up, dull, and cool. We frequently become more delicate to commotion as we age, and light and intensity can likewise cause rest issues. Utilizing a sound machine, ear plugs, or a rest veil can help.

Guarantee your bed is agreeable. Utilizing a movable base, for instance, can help both your upper and lower body, give rest apnea

ETERNAL VITALITY

alleviation, and diminish back torment as you age.

Utilize your room just for rest and sex. By not working, staring at the television, or involving your PC in bed, your cerebrum will connect the room with simply rest and sex.

Move room takes off of view. The light can disturb your rest and tensely watching the minutes tick by is a dependable recipe for sleep deprivation.

Tip 3: Keep a standard sleep time schedule

Keep a predictable rest plan. Hit the hay and wake up at similar times consistently, even on ends of the week.

ETERNAL VITALITY

Shut out wheezing. On the off chance that wheezing is keeping you up, attempt earplugs, a background noise, or separate rooms.

Hit the hay before. Change your sleep time to match when you want to hit the hay, regardless of whether that is sooner than it used to be.

Foster alleviating sleep time customs. Washing up, playing music, or rehearsing an unwinding strategy like moderate muscle unwinding, care reflection, or profound breathing can assist you with slowing down before bed.

Limit tranquilizers and dozing pills. Many tranquilizers make side impacts and are not implied for long haul use. Resting pills don't address the reasons for a sleeping disorder and might exacerbate it over the long haul.

Join sex and rest. Sex and actual closeness, like embracing, can prompt tranquil rest.

Tip 4: Gain proficiency with the most effective ways to rest

In the event that you don't feel completely alert during the day, a rest might give the energy you really want to perform completely until the end of the day. Examination to check whether it helps you.

A few ways to rest:

Keep it short. Rests as short as five minutes can further develop readiness and certain memory processes. A great many people benefit from restricting rests to 15-45 minutes. You might feel sluggish and incapable to think after a more extended rest.

Rest early. Rest promptly in the early evening. Resting past the point of no return in the day might disturb your evening time rest.

Be agreeable. Attempt to rest in an agreeable climate ideally with restricted light and clamor.

Tip 5: Use diet to further develop rest as you age

As well as eating a rest accommodating eating routine during the day, it's especially critical to watch what you put in your body some time before sleep time.

Limit caffeine late in the day. Stay away from espresso, tea, pop, and chocolate late in the day.

Stay away from liquor before sleep time. It could appear to be that liquor makes you languid, however it will really disturb your rest.

Fulfill your yearning preceding bed. Have a light tidbit like low-sugar cereal, yogurt, or warm milk.

Eliminate sweet food varieties. Eating an eating routine high in sugar and refined carbs like white bread, white rice, pasta, and French fries can cause alertness around evening time and haul you out of the profound, supportive phases of rest.

Stay away from huge feasts or fiery food sources not long before sleep time. Indigestion or discomfort may result from large or spicy meals. Attempt to have an unassuming size supper no less than 3 hours before sleep time.

Limit fluid admission before rest. Limit what you drink inside the 90 minutes before sleep time to restrict how frequently you awaken to utilize the washroom around evening time.

Tip 6: Practice for defeating rest issues in more seasoned grown-ups

ETERNAL VITALITY

Practice — particularly high-impact movement — discharges synthetic compounds in your body that advance more relaxing rest. Regardless of whether you have portability issues, there are endless exercises you can do to set yourself up for a decent night's rest. In any case, consistently counsel your primary care physician prior to leaving on any new work out schedule.

Try:

Swimming/water works out. Swimming laps is a delicate method for developing wellness and is perfect for sore joints or feeble muscles. Numerous people group and YMCA pools have swim programs only for more established grown-ups, as well as water-based practice classes.

Dancing. Take a dance class or go dancing if you enjoy moving to music. Dance classes are likewise an extraordinary method for broadening your interpersonal organization.

Yard bowling, bocce, or pétanque. These ball games are delicate ways of working out. The more you walk, and the brisker the speed, the more high-impact benefit you'll insight.

Golfing. Another exercise that doesn't require a lot of movement is golf. Strolling adds an oxygen consuming reward and investing energy in the course with companions can work on your temperament.

ETERNAL VITALITY

Cycling or running. Assuming you are looking great, you can run and cycle until late throughout everyday life. Both can be done outside or on a treadmill or stationary bike.

ETERNAL VITALITY

CHAPTER SIX
WAY OF LIFE ELEMENTS

Pressure The board

"Everyone encounters pressure," ,previous long-term overseer of health at Judson and individual from Judson's directorate. " It's the body's normal response to an improvement or stressor that upsets our physical or mental harmony. It's additionally generally known as our 'survival' reaction."

This reaction to critical circumstances served us well in the developmental cycle, permitting us to adjust and get by in risky circumstances.

Here is your body's physiological reaction to this kind of pressure:

ETERNAL VITALITY

Expanded pulse and heartbeat

Elevated muscle readiness/strain

Expanded pulse

Quick relaxing

Stomach related framework lull

Resistant framework concealment

Elevated feeling of readiness/absence of rest

Expansion in cortisol creation (stress chemical)

You can perceive how these responses can be useful in risky circumstances. Our body, in exceptional style, answers so the fundamental capabilities for guaranteed endurance are upgraded. Really noteworthy, truly. In any case, when the hazardous circumstance died down, our body was intended to get back to homeostasis.

The issue we're finding in the present culture is that a significant number of us have this "survival" component turned on constantly all through our lives, and in regular circumstances that don't warrant this degree of reaction. Allude back to the rundown above, and envision those responses being somebody's general condition.

Chronic exposure to this kind of stress over the course of our lives can result in subpar

ETERNAL VITALITY

performance and the breakdown of various internal organs, down to the cellular level.

Scientists have recognized normal medical issues related with persistent pressure:

Coronary illness

Diabetes

Migraines

Asthma

Wretchedness

Nervousness

Gastrointestinal Issues

Alzheimer's Illness

ETERNAL VITALITY

As may be obvious, these are issues that don't influence just more seasoned grown-ups, however the individuals from each age.

So what can really be done? How can we reduce our stress and live a full and healthy life? Your life's stressors probably won't ever go away completely. Yet, we can figure out how to control our responses to ease our "survival" reaction, consequently relieving the adverse consequences of weight on the body.

5 Methods for lessening Pressure

1.) Care

A feeling of care is one of our essential method for managing pressure, as per Sara Peckham. To calm a bustling psyche and become more mindful of the current second means we're less up to speed previously and we decrease our concern for what's in store. We're ready to appreciate "the at this point" while as yet recognizing and tolerating our sentiments and considerations.

"Contemplation is a fundamental means to accomplishing care and lessening pressure," Science is finding out about the cerebrum's capacity to adjust and revamp during contemplation. The term for this is "brain plasticity." Consider "attention" to be a muscle; Through meditation, you can exercise it, and it will get stronger.

ETERNAL VITALITY

Notwithstanding stress and uneasiness, a significant number of us go to the marvels of present day medication and get an energizer or hostile to tension drug from our PCP. This won't take care of the issue; all things being equal, it will just veil its side effects. Instead, mindfulness will assist you in getting to the source.

2.) Work out

Notwithstanding actual advantages like expanding lung limit, bone thickness and generally life span, practice particularly affects mind wellbeing. Furthermore, in light of the fact that this is where a large portion of our pressure starts, exercise's effect on diminishing feelings of anxiety couldn't possibly be more significant.

A study that was carried out at the University of Illinois made it abundantly clear that engaging in moderate but consistent aerobic exercise can improve our overall cognitive health. More established grown-ups who partook in the review went for 40-minute strolls three days out of each week throughout the span of one year.

In that year alone, the members saw a two-percent increment in the size of their hippocampus, the region of the mind engaged with memory and learning. Conversely, without work out, more established grown-ups can hope to see a decline in the size of their hippocampus by around a couple of percent every year.

Practice spikes the age of new synapses - this is currently indisputable reality. Yet, how much activity do we want? Not however much you could think.

The Rush Memory and Maturing Venture, directed in 2012 in Chicago with in excess of 1,200 elderly folks taking part, obviously exhibited that, as Dr. Perlmutter references in his book Grain Cerebrum: ". . . we can't misjudge the force of minimal expense, effectively available, and aftereffect free exercises that may not involve formal activity.

ETERNAL VITALITY

The simple activities of day to day living can give cerebrum defensive advantages at whatever stage in life."

3.) Body Control

Notwithstanding conventional activity like strolling, heart stimulating exercise or power lifting, there exist more unpretentious types of what we'll call "body control" that can significantly affect lessening feelings of anxiety. The short rundown incorporates treatments and projects that are accessible at Judson:

Judo

Yoga

ETERNAL VITALITY

Knead

Craniosacral Treatment

Reiki

The advantages of these treatments and activities include:

Enhancing mental capacity and concentration Improving conditions like Alzheimer's, multiple sclerosis, and Parkinson's These activities, in conjunction with other forms of physical exercise, assist people of all ages in maintaining independence and increasing their sense of mindfulness. They also help to accumulate energy by releasing endorphins (rather than depleting it).

ETERNAL VITALITY

Numerous exercises like yoga and Jujitsu are for the most part of a bigger program or exist in a class structure. This has the additional advantage of uniting individuals and empowering a feeling of local area, which is our fourth method for assisting you with lessening pressure.

4.) A Feeling of Local area

"As we age, regularly we lose sharpness, vision, hearing, and in some cases memory," " Physically, we also have more to deal with; what's more, as these things occur, we will quite often segregate ourselves since we would rather not be 'found out.'"

ETERNAL VITALITY

This is the specific inverse of what we ought to do, and upheld by various logical examinations. A feeling of local area and warm connections are basic to our physical and emotional well-being from early stages

5.) Eat Healthfully Thick Food sources and Stay away from Sugar

A less generally realized stressor comes as food varieties lacking nourishing thickness.

In the present society it's very much simple to eat food sources that are almost absent any and all nourishment. Drive-through joints are at each significant convergence - and in the event that not you'll frequently find rather a pharmacy loaded to the roof with potato chips, sweet tidbits and refined staples.

In a time when it is well known that Americans are gaining weight, experiencing chronic pain, and dying from conditions associated with severe cognitive impairments at an increasing rate, we cannot ignore the role that poor diets play.

Also, sustenance's effect on the mind couldn't possibly be more significant. It's basic to our psychological wellness and feelings of anxiety that the food we eat be stuffed with nutrients and minerals our bodies need to work ideally. This for the most part implies an eating routine low in carbs and high in solid, soaked fats. Suggested consumes less calories incorporate an overflow of vegetables, fish, meat, poultry, nuts, eggs and mixed greens.

Furthermore, on the off chance that you do nothing else healthfully to decrease your pressure, maybe the #1 proposal we can make is this: Keep away from SUGAR.

Sugar's impact on the body is just negative; notwithstanding, it's simple energy, which is the reason so many of us desire it. However, excessive sugar consumption is directly linked to obesity, diabetes, disease, and even death. On the off chance that we can remove sugar totally, we'd find that quite a bit of our pressure and tension just disappears, notwithstanding a summary of other medical advantages like directed circulatory strain levels, expanded mineral substance in your body, and expanded mental capability.

Social Associations and Aging

It is critical to solid maturing. Studies have shown that more established individuals who have close associations and connections live longer, yet in addition adapt better to medical issue and experience less discouragement. Life advances can influence the number and nature of individuals' social and local area organizations. For instance, loved ones might move away, which can adversely affect somebody's informal organization. However, a progress, for example, the introduction of another relative can bring positive changes.

What are a portion of the existence conditions that can influence one's social connectedness?

Changes in one's health as well as one's ability to walk and get around Changes in one's job and income Changes in one's housing situation Changes in one's family and friends, particularly one's spouse Challenges with getting to work While driving is as of now not a choice, separation turns into a huge issue, particularly in networks where there is practically zero public transportation.

Here are some proactive steps you can take to stay connected and avoid loneliness.

ETERNAL VITALITY

Participate in Community Events. Contemplate exercises you appreciate and check out your local area for ways of reaching out. Consider the neighborhood Y, a public venue, or a nearby spot of love.

Volunteer. Not exclusively will chipping in help your local area, it is an extraordinary chance to meet new individuals.

Utilize technology. It may not always be possible to meet a friend in person. Find a workable pace on innovation since there are different ways of conveying and keep in contact with your friends and family. Share pictures through email or web-based entertainment. Have a video discussion on your PC or by downloading an application on your cell phone! (Look at The Eldercare Finder's handout on Innovation Choices for More established Grown-ups for more tech tips.).

Attempt Elective Treatments. Think about owning a pet. Walking a pet is a great way to meet new people and there are many adult animals in need of a new home. Dive deeper into the advantages of back rub and fragrance based treatment and afterward attempt it!

Think about Various Lodging. It might be sensible to weigh the benefits and drawbacks of changing places or living arrangements so that there are more chances to meet new people and socialize with them.

Be Dynamic. Not exclusively is active work imperative in forestalling falls, it is an astonishing method for meeting others.

ETERNAL VITALITY

CONCLUSION

In this present reality where media frequently likens youth with excellence, it's not difficult to feel eclipsed as we experience the regular maturing process. Notwithstanding, this story doesn't mirror the genuine experience of endless ladies...

Many have imparted to us their excursion of feeling more enabled, certain, and alluring as they embrace their full grown years. This, we accept, is the substance of genuine excellence.

All in all, how might you commend your developing magnificence in a culture zeroed in on youth?

Six suggestions are discussed in this article.

ETERNAL VITALITY

Tip #1: Careful Media Utilization

Our lives are immersed with screens - telephones, workstations, tablets. These steady media collaborations can slant our impression of magnificence.

Despite its difficulties, limiting screen time is essential. The people who connect less with media frequently end up more associated with their inward satisfaction and excellence, liberated from unreasonable guidelines.

Keep in mind, internal satisfaction shows and even surpasses outer appearances.

Tip #2: Develop Positive Associations

ETERNAL VITALITY

The assessments of those we hold dear can profoundly influence our self-view. Encircle yourself with people who perceive and commend the excellence of development. Their encouraging words can have a big impact on how you see yourself and help you keep a healthy perspective on getting older.

At the point when in discussion, in the event that you hear cynicism about maturing, assist with changing the tone to a positive one, while as yet understanding and being sympathetic of others' encounters.

Tip #3: Redefine Makeup Use

Numerous corrective brands advance covering the normal indications of maturing. However, a more gainful methodology is utilizing cosmetics to complement your regular highlights.

Embrace it as a tool for enhancement, not concealment. This shift in perspective can significantly boost self-appreciation. It will change how you apply makeup and think about yourself every day.

Tip #4: Use Skincare as Self Care

With the best ingredients, focus your skincare on loving and taking care of yourself. It ought to be less about appearance, and more about the wellbeing and feel of your skin. Selecting natural, normal items lines up with this concentration to adore yourself and backing your skin's wellbeing.

In the end, healthy skin will naturally radiate beauty.

Tip #5: Enrich Mind and Soul

Embrace exercises that feed your psyche and soul, encouraging a more profound identity mindfulness and internal harmony. This can include mindfulness practices, meditation, journaling, or engaging in creative pursuits like painting or writing.

These practices not just add to mental and close to home prosperity yet in addition develop a more profound association with yourself, improving confidence and appreciation for the world as you age.

Tip #6: Care for Your Physical Body

Integrate a balance of physical activity, mindful eating, and restful sleep into your daily routine. Rehearses like yoga, nature strolls, or delicate outside practices offer a double advantage: they care for your actual prosperity while at the same time enhancing your brain and soul. Such an all encompassing way to deal with wellbeing supports your general wellbeing as well as transmits a dynamic, positive energy that is noticeable remotely. The genuine quintessence of excellence far outperforms the bounds old

ETERNAL VITALITY

enough. It's an ever-evolving tapestry woven from confidence, radiance, and a deep-seated comfort in one's own skin.

As we journey through life, each year adds to our story, bringing with it a unique blend of grace, wisdom, and strength. These qualities contribute to a beauty that is both timeless and profound.

Allow us then to rethink the norms of excellence, not as a benchmark to be accomplished in youth, however as a continuous festival of our life's process. It's about honoring the laughter lines as much as the youthful glow, cherishing the wisdom in our eyes as much as the smoothness of skin.

Eternal Vitality

This viewpoint enables us to embrace each phase of our existence with happiness and pride. Together, we should support another account of excellence - one that commends the polish inborn in development, perceives the charm in experience, and finds the wonder in becoming older. In doing as such, we elevate ourselves as well as set a lively, positive model for a long time into the future. Reversing time is not what defines beauty; it's tied in with carrying on with our best life at each second, praising every year for the extraordinary gifts it brings.